ALZHEIMER
My Love

A Play By
SAL ATLANTIS PHOENIX

Copyright © 2024 by Sal Atlantis Phoenix.

ISBN: 9798890904164 (sc)
ISBN: 9798890904171 (e)

All rights reserved. No part of this book may be reproduced or transmitted in any form or by any means, electronic or mechanical, including photocopying, recording, or by any information storage and retrieval system, without permission in writing from the copyright owner.

EXPRESSO
Executive Center 777, Dunsmuir Street Vancouver, BC V71K4
1-888-721-0662 ext 101
info@expressopublishing.com

FIRST LEAD: JOSEPH
SECOND LEAD: MARY
THIRD LEAD: DOCTOR ALLEN

MAIN CHARACTERS:

JOSEPH: IN HIS LATE SIXTIES, EMOTIONALLY DEVASTATED AND FRUSTRATED BY HIS WIFE'S ALZHEIMER'S DISEASE.

MARY: IN HER LATE SIXTIES, SUFFERING FROM DEVASTATING ALZHEIMER'S DISEASE. **DOCTOR ALLEN:** MEDICAL DOCTOR

AUXILIARY CHARACTERS: COMPANION JUDY AND HER FIANCÉ.

BASIC STORY LINE: MARY AND JOSEPH ARE BELOVED COUPLES WHO HAVE GONE THROUGH THE LIFE'S CHALLENGING JOURNEY. JOSEPH IS DESPERATE.

SCENE SYNOPSIS: THE PERFORMANCE OF THE PLAY HAPPENS IN A PARK AND IN JOSEPH'S HOME IN MANHATTAN.

ACT I
EARLY STAGE OF ALZHEIMER'S

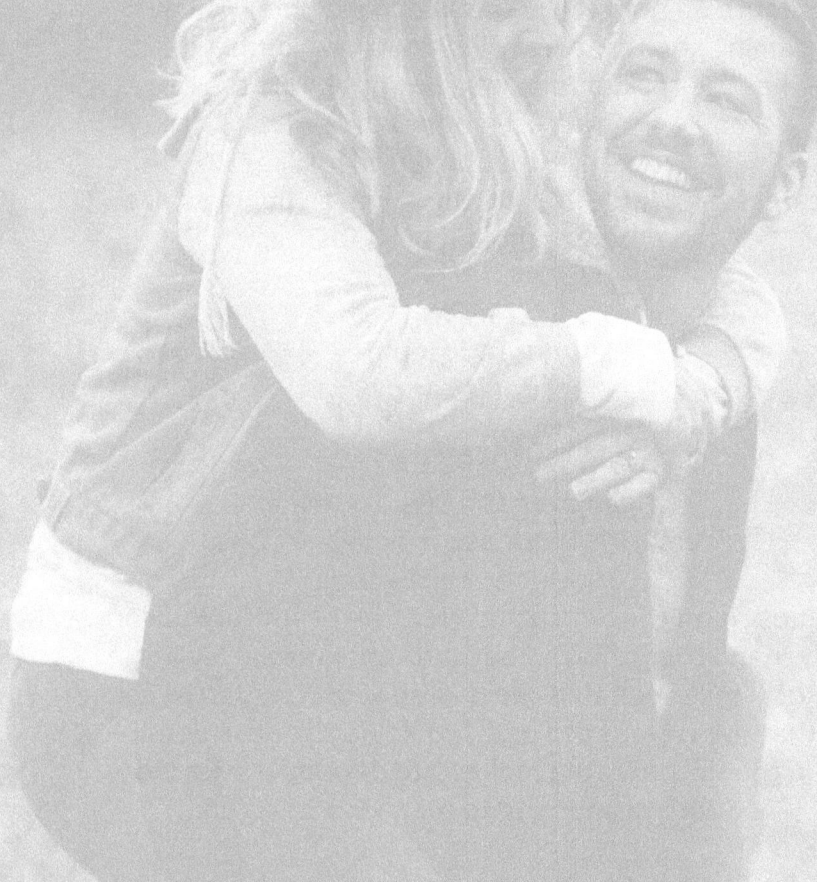

SCENE 1

IN THE BACKGROUND SCENE, VIEW OF THE HUDSON RIVER AND GEORGE WASHINGTON BRIDGE. THE BENCH IS TWO STEPS ABOVE THE PATH WAY AND IS SURROUNDED BY GREEN TREES. ALONG THE EDGE OF THE PATHWAY, BEAUTIFUL SPRING FLOWERS BLOOM. A COUPLE HOLDING HANDS ENTER AND WALK SLOWLY AND STOP TO LOOK ADMIRINGLY AT THE FLOWERS.

JOSEPH
Spring flowers are like youth. They are at the beginning stage of life, full of dreams and glorious expectations. Youth do not realize that old man winter will be coming soon, and he will shroud the youth. Youth has the spirit of eternity, but not in the reality.
(pause, lean forward)
Look at that beautiful iris.
(caress iris gently, look at Mary with a cunning smile)
Do you mind if I kiss iris?

MARY
(ignore Joseph)
I don't care.

JOSEPH
(lean over and kiss the iris)
Of course, iris is not as attractive as you are.
(motion to the bench)
Let us sit on the bench and view the beautiful Hudson River and the Palisades beyond. You know... My uncle Rockefeller donated the palisades to New Jersey so that the view of the park would not be obstructed in the future by the real estate developers. He did not donate anything to me... Son of a gun...

MARY
Don't be childish.

JOSEPH
I wish Rockefeller was my uncle...
(gesture to the bench)
Let us go and sit on the bench. Mary,
hold on to me... Be careful.

Directions
(Joseph holds Mary's arm and directs her up
the steps to the bench. She loses balance as she
walks up, and he holds her by the waist and helps
her to sit on the bench. He sits next to her)

JOSEPH
Do you remember this bench?

MARY
(irritated)
What do you mean?

JOSEPH
I mean... How did this bench flourish our lives?

MARY
Don't be ridiculous.

JOSEPH
Do you remember? We met on this bench!
(sigh)
I remember well... I was walking, lost in my thoughts,
and I saw a charming woman sitting on the bench and
reading a book and writing notes. I thought maybe
I should sit next to her and get her opinion.

MARY
Get opinion about what?

JOSEPH
Well... It was about how to establish my life... I was arriving at middle age, and it was time to structure my life. I was not young anymore. Rebellious days were over. It turned out to be that I was a rebel without a cause. I believed in 'Power to the People'. The reality was 'dollar to the people'. I was very naïve and politically incorrect.
(thoughtful)
I had to conform to the establishment. Especially that time when I lost my job during the recession, and I was trying to survive on the unemployment benefits. In the old days, unemployment benefits would last for twenty-four months. Now, in this present economic recession, unemployment benefits last only three months. Conservatives accused the liberals as socialist and reduced the benefits. I don't know who is right or wrong. I can only tell that guys like me always pay the price for the economic collapse.

MARY
(serious)
Conservatives should be blamed!

JOSEPH
I am surprised that you were concentrating!

MARY
What do you mean?... Of course, I was concentrating... Am I stupid?!

JOSEPH
Of course not... Once in a while you get confused and forget things... It may be the 'senior moments' or, the beginning of a more serious condition.

MARY
What do you mean by 'more serious condition'?

JOSEPH
I mean... You know... Your mother died of Alzheimer's disease and your brother died of some form of neurological disease. It is in the family!

MARY
(agitated)
I am fine... I am good. Medical gene inheritance theory is ridiculous. My aunt did not have Alzheimer's, and she was as sharp as can be until her death.

JOSEPH
Of course, you are good, darling. But you should get a checkup with a neurologist to make sure that you are good. I always get an annual checkup. I am a cancer survivor because early detection saved my life.

MARY
(angrily stand and walk down the steps)
I am going home. I don't need anybody's help. I am independent. I can take care of myself.

JOSEPH
Mary, do you remember, three months ago, you walked out and got lost? I had to call the police. It took them eight hours to find you. They found you walking alone on the East River drive. You walked one hundred twelve blocks late in the evening.
(talk to self)
What is the point of trying to communicate! The damn Alzheimer's disease is incurable.
(get up and rush down the steps to grab her)
Relax darling. It is too early to go home.
(pull her up the steps and sit her on the bench)

I am so grateful that I met you in the park. You
steered my life in the right direction.

MARY
(confused)
What did I do?

JOSEPH
You encouraged me to be an educator. That was the
right job for me. It was better and satisfying for me to
communicate with the kids rather than the adults. You were
good and dedicated worker better than me, I must admit!

MARY
My mother was a good and dedicated worker.
She did take care of me and my brother and the
elderly people in the neighborhood. She loved
to help people. She had enormous energy.

JOSEPH
When did you notice the symptoms of her Alzheimer's illness?

MARY
My mother began talking and repeating about the same
thing. She was misplacing things at home. She would go
out to shopping and come back without the shopping cart.
She wouldn't remember where she left the cart. I rented
a one-bedroom apartment in my building and moved
her in. She needed supervision. One day, she walked out
and did not come back. She was lost. I called the police,
and they found her walking ten miles away from home.
I realized I couldn't handle her anymore. I sent her to a
nursing home. I used to go to see her after work once
a week to make sure that she was taken care of. After
returning home, I would cry. (pause, begin to cry)
If I get Alzheimer's disease, I will jump down the window
and kill myself... I don't want to live with that disease.

JOSEPH
(lean back on the bench, take a deep breath and gently hold her hand and kiss her on the cheek, try to comfort her)
Please don't cry. I understand your feelings, although personal tragedy is not devastating to the third person as it is for the beloved... Now I realize that I should have been more helpful and emotionally supportive to you.

Directions
(Mary continues sobbing. Joseph puts his other arm on her shoulder and pulls her close to him. On the background screen, a picture of a three-year old girl appears. Joseph looks at the little girl and smiles at her. He tries to distract Mary's sorrow by trying to get her attention to focus on the child)

JOSEPH
Look at that little one. Isn't she pretty?

MARY
(wipe off tear with hand and look at the child)
She is beautiful. She is beautiful. I love her... I love her...

JOSEPH
Little girl is pretty like you when you were a child.

MARY
When I was at her age, they wanted me to be a model. My father did not agree.

JOSEPH
Why not?

MARY
In the old days, modeling was not a lucrative career.

JOSEPH
(look at the child with an inquisitive expression)
How old are you, little girl?

Directions
(backstage sound of the child stuttering:
'I am four years old')

JOSEPH
You are younger than I.
(imitate childish stutter)
I am five years old.

Directions
(child stutters 'No')

JOSEPH
How old do you think I am?

Directions
(The child stutters 'Ten')

JOSEPH
Thank you, darling.
(jokes)
No objections, your honor!

MARY
(interferes)
Joseph, don't be childish!

JOSEPH
Why not? Childhood is the best years of human life. My mother did tell me the same thing. (sad expression)

She would say 'son you are joking all the time. You are like a little kid. People won't take you seriously. Grow up, son!' I would reply and tell her, 'Mommy, I don't wan't to grow up! I want to be your little baby. If I grow up, I will be dealing with the doctors, lawyers, politicians, and the businessmen. I want to be a little baby and hug in your arms eternally.'

MARY
(look at the child)
I love you… I will take you home… I love you… I love you…

Directions
(female voice echoes in the background: 'Sheila, where are you… I am waiting for you. Hurry up, come back…' Little girl screams: 'Mommy, I am here… I am here, mommy' The picture of the child fades)

MARY
Joseph, did you have children?

JOSEPH
We did not have children!

MARY
(depressed)
Why did we not have children?

JOSEPH
We could have, but we didn't want to have children… I don't know why? Do you know why?

MARY
(resentful)
It was your fault…

JOSEPH
It was not my fault! You were too busy taking care of your mother in the nursing home. Now I realize how painful to be a caregiver to an Alzheimer's patient; especially if she is the loved one! We were not young anymore... and your job was your priority... I must admit, my jobs were always secondary responsibility to me. Maybe that is why I was never successful. MARY. You were strange. You did not express your love to me.

JOSEPH
Yes, darling, you are right. But I loved you. I was always an introvert and you were an extrovert.

MARY
(nervous)
You always left me alone and went to see your mother. Your mother was more important to you.

JOSEPH
Darling! Mothers are the true lovers of the sons. Without my mother, I wouldn't exist.

MARY
I knew I was not your true love. You were uncommitted. Why should I have your child!...

JOSEPH
Our child!...

MARY
Whatever...

JOSEPH
I always believed in you. You were smarter than I. That's for sure!... I wanted you to make the decision. Because we were not married, having a child, without marriage would

be very irresponsible. I was assuming that you were deeply in love with me and you would persuade me to have a child.

MARY

Having a child without marrying you would put me in social and psychological burden... Why did you not commit yourself to a permanent relation with me? Why did you leave me and go away every summer to see your mother and stay with her for months?

JOSEPH

My mother was old. I left her alone. I was concerned, and I felt guilty. Mother's love can't be replaced, you know...
(serious)
She was concerned about my future. Like every mother, she wanted me to have children... I knew that having a child is like love and marriage. It can be heavenly or inferno, depending on the personality. When we are young, we are more concerned to raising a child because of challenging and sometimes frustrating responsibilities. As we get older, we have different perspective. Seeing children brings back life to us.
(feel guilty, try to justify)
I wanted you to make a decision. I said to myself, 'if Mary wants to have our child even though we are not married, she must be in love with me'. In that case, I will marry her and settle down'.

MARY

(alert and frustrated look at Joseph angrily)
I was one month pregnant. I gave you
a hint. You did not respond!

JOSEPH

I told you I wanted you to make the decision. I wanted to find out if you were in love with me and commit your life to our relation... What was your decision?

MARY
(turn face around and pause)
I had an abortion.

JOSEPH
(lean head forward, hold it with both hands and begin to sob)
Oh, God! Why was I so irresponsible?... Why was I so simple-minded?... Why did you not bestow providence on me?...

MARY
(slowly get up from the bench and walk down the steps and head towards the flowers. Caress the flowers and murmur)
Beautiful babies... I love you... I love you...

JOSEPH
(stand up and slowly walk towards her, hold her hands, draw her in and kiss her on the forehead)
Life is a challenging journey. Especially for guys like me who predict their own future covered by illusion instead of foreseeing the reality. They pay the price and their life is a vicious cycle... Mary darling, let us enjoy the moment whether it is rain or sunshine. Every day is a bonus day! They should teach the reality in schools instead of math and science. Eventually, everyone can learn math and science after hard work. But when you learn the reality of life, it is too late to recover the lost days... life goes on... We should forgive and forget!

MARY
(kiss Joseph passionately)
I love you...

JOSEPH
(sing)
Mary my love
Whatever will be, will be
Our future is not ours to see...

Our future is in the hands of the MD...
Que sera... sera

MARY
What do you mean by MD?

JOSEPH
Darling... I was singing. They say singing and
music is good therapy to improve memory.

MARY
That is medical doctors' nonsense opinion.

JOSEPH
I agree darling. Doctors are like politicians.
They try to calm the people with statements
if they can't find medical treatment.

Directions
(the sound of the children laughing and
shouting is heard in the background)

JOSEPH
Darling, we should go to midtown and do something.
We should keep our mind busy. We are retired, and we
have to be mentally active to avoid old age dementia.

MARY
(agitated and in denial of her onset dementia)
Why are you referring to dementia all the time? I am good...
I am good... (start pacing up and down nervously)

JOSEPH
(follow her, try to divert her attention)
Remember darling... We used to go to Columbus Circle
and walk through the Central Park to the East Side and
sit on the bench and watch the swans in the lake and

watch them move through the water gracefully. The young generation would lie on the grass to tan, and the tourists would walk by, taking pictures of the park and the high-rise modern and classic architectural buildings overlooking the park... Do you remember the Plaza Hotel where we had dinner after we got married in Staten Island?...

MARY
(confused)
What do you mean?... I mean... When did it happen?...

JOSEPH
Do you remember?... We went to the City Clerk's Office in downtown Manhattan and there was a long line of couples waiting to get married. You didn't want to wait too long. So I asked the clerk for another location, and he told me that at this time of the day the only place that would not be crowded would be the Staten Island Borough Clerk's office. We picked up our car from the garage nearby, and I drove to Staten Island, and we said to the Judge 'until death do us apart'... You see, that is why I am with you always, even though you may have a medical condition...

MARY
(annoyed)
What do you mean by 'I may have a medical condition'!... Stop the nonsense...

JOSEPH
I mean... You know... I mean 'the old age condition'... Happens to all of us... After the wedding, we drove over the Verrazano Bridge and had dinner at the Plaza Hotel. Across from us, Senator Kerry was dining with his wife... He was a presidential candidate for the coming election year. I went to his table and said, 'Senator Kerry, I want to express my gratitude to you for your courage. Years ago,

when you returned from Vietnam, I remember seeing you on television during a Senate investigation about the Vietnam War and, as a Vietnam War Veteran, you were challenging the justification of the war'. We shook hands and I returned to our table and celebrated our marriage... Each time I walk by the Plaza Hotel, I realize that time goes by too fast... I remember the days when life seemed to be challenging when I was young; in reality, every day is a bonus day because life is too short... When I was working, I was enthusiastic about the end of the work on Friday. Saturdays and Sundays were youthful days of excitement and venture... As I get older, I realize that another week diminished from my life at the end of the week and it is not refundable.

MARY
What are you going do about it?

JOSEPH
Nothing really, except enjoy every moment whether it is rain or sunshine... Maybe we should go to The Lincoln Center to see a performance. We can go early in the afternoon and see the young teenagers coming out of school, wondering around the pool in the Lincoln Plaza; some of them laying on the grass on the miniature slope across the pool and joking and laughing at each other. It brings back youthful life to me...

MARY
You mean artificial youthful life!...

JOSEPH
Yes... It is better than death... Darling, let us be positive... What about going to the Village and going to the New York University students' theater or musical performance?... Afterward, we can wander around in the Washington Square.

Directions
(Mary ignores Joseph. She does not respond. Joseph is persistent. Tries to get Mary's attention)

JOSEPH
Remember, you had lots of energy and you were a good walker. We used to walk on Madison Avenue from forty-second street to fifty-nine street and observe every fashion store... And then we would walk west to Fifth Avenue and walk north along the upper-class high society neighborhood... I used to dream about living among the Fifth Avenue high society... Now I realize that living in good health in Harlem and surrounded by loving big family is a better choice than being lonely, unhealthy and old and living in the high-class Fifth Avenue society... Would you like to go to the Metropolitan Museum today?

MARY
(uncomfortable, walk away from Joseph)
No, I don't want to go. You go by yourself.

JOSEPH
Darling, I feel nostalgic and depressed when I walk alone by myself. Too many memories flash back about the good old youthful days. Together, we used to explore the culture and the life in the city.
(smile, open arms, look at her and sing)
Give me Manhattan,
Manhattan only
Peter Minuet bought Manhattan for me
So that I could meet thee...

MARY
You are childish... Why are you singing?

JOSEPH
Darling, I am singing because singing
is good therapy for dementia.

MARY
(very agitated, scream)
Stop that... I don't like you... I am good...
I don't have any dementia problem... I am
independent... I can live on my own. If you don't
want to live with me go back to your mother.

JOSEPH
Don't you remember... My mother passed away!

MARY
When did she die?

JOSEPH
Six years ago.

Directions
(Mary looks blank. No response. Joseph
tries to stimulate her memory)

JOSEPH
Unfortunately, your mother and your brother also passed
away. I was sad when you called me and told me that our
mother passed away, and you could not come to visit my
mother when I was visiting her during the summer vacation.

MARY
(suddenly alert, look at Joseph and
begin to converse diligently)
When my mother died, I cried. I was devastated. I made the
funeral arrangement and buried her next to my father, who
died twenty years before from lung cancer. He was a heavy
smoker. After her burial, I suddenly felt relieved. I felt guilty.

I was expecting to cry for days. I did not. Then I realized that taking care of her for eighteen years had a psychological impact on me. Mentally, I was in prison. Even when I sent her to a nursing home, no matter what, going and seeing her in an environment of destitute made me desperate. (pause, lost in thoughts, look blank at distance)

JOSEPH
I understand your feelings, darling. I am so sorry for what you have gone through.

MARY
You were not with your mother when she was old and died. Your sister took care of her. She carried the burden.

JOSEPH
That is true. But I had the responsibility of my father.

MARY
What do you mean by 'responsibility'?...
You were not living with him!...

JOSEPH
Yes, that is true. He was living alone. But I used to visit him often, even I had to quit my job because they would not give me permission to get extra days off. He was politically incorrect, and he was on the black list. He ended up in Paris, believing that it would be a more liberal and permissive place to live. He was naïve, like me!... He didn't realize that this world was the same old, same old world... Money speaks, not the idealism... He died in Paris. His official death certificate indicates heart failure. According to some unofficial sources, his death was man made rather than nature made, which was imposed on the politically incorrect naïve individuals. His friends were afraid to send his body home. They wanted to bury him in Paris. I objected and wanted him to be buried in his hometown. I believed that his

compatriots would not forget him. I doubt if they bother to visit his grave anymore. I was so naïve... Once you are gone, you are gone!... The only legacy that remains is the legacy of the "Almighty Dollar"... That is the real human history...
(silent, expression very sad, take a
deep breath and look at Mary)
Your brother's death was sudden. I thought he would live longer... His wife called you and told you that he had a stroke, and he was dying. We rushed to see him. He was in bed. You sat by him, talked to him quietly, and caressed him. He looked at you and mumbled incomprehensible words from time to time. Then you cried and asked me to sit next to him and told me to hold his hand. His wife must have informed your brother's first wife about his condition. When I was in the room sitting by him, your brother's first wife walked in and looked at him briefly. She said 'Hi, how are you doing Michael?'... Michael looked at her with a smile and mumbled. His first wife looked at me and said nervously, 'He is going to die,' and walked out... (look at Mary and try to get her involved in the conversation to stimulate her memory) Do you remember his burial?

MARY
(do not respond)

JOSEPH
His wife Peggy decided to bury him on Long Island. It was a long ride from Manhattan. On his gravestone 'Vietnam' was carved... I did not ask why she had that word carved on. I was curious... When Michael was in the air force briefly; I wonder if he was involved in secret missions!... I know that Peggy was conservative Republican and supported the Vietnam War. Anyhow... Bygones are bygones... Life goes on... Past is past... War and peace are historical twins... Two years after Michael's death, poor Peggy died of brain hemorrhage.

MARY
(suddenly alert)
My aunt Nonie also died.

JOSEPH
Oh, you remembered!...

MARY
Of course, I remember... I am good...

JOSEPH
Of course darling, you remember... I don't think
your aunt was impressed with me. She liked
accomplished man... I must admit I was not

MARY
She was not impressed with you because you did not commit
yourself to a permanent relation with me while she was alive!

JOSEPH
Unfortunately, I did not make an early commitment.
Now I realize it was poor judgment. Maybe it was
lack of my intelligence... But I was faithful to you
during our relation and after our marriage.
(agitated)
Were you faithful to me?

Directions
(Mary avoids him, turns her face the other way and does
not respond. Joseph grabs her arm and shakes her. Holds
her face, turns it around towards him and screams)

JOSEPH
Were you faithful to me?

MARY
(do not respond)

JOSEPH
I knew you were very affectionate and caring, wanted to help people and you had a domineering personality. You wanted to be in charge of everyone. You wanted attention. You wanted to be in control. That is what I thought. Now, I realize that I had poor judgment. (agitated)
Did you have an affair with my classmate?

MARY
(ignore Joseph and look the other way)

JOSEPH
(scream)
Did you have an affair with my classmate?

MARY
(look blank)
Which one?

JOSEPH
The one who works as a secret agent for the 'Big Brothers'. He came to see me and stayed with us. I suspected that he was checking on me to see if I would get involved in 'politically incorrect activities'. I didn't question him. I told you that his parents were divorced and he had a difficult life. Because of that, I thought you felt sympathetic and wanted to establish an affectionate relation with him.

Directions
(Mary does not respond, turns her face the other way and looks blank. Joseph holds her face and turns around towards him with force)

MARY
(scream)
You are hurting me.

JOSEPH
Yes, I am hurting you, but you are breaking my heart...
Did you have an affair with your cousin when he
stayed with us and when you went to visit him?

MARY
(rebut)
Were you faithful to me?

JOSEPH
Yes... I was faithful to you!...

MARY
Why?...

JOSEPH
Why?... Because I believed that I had to have compassion and loving relation with a female before I would commit myself to her. That relation doesn't happen overnight. Just having sex is inadequate for me... I would rather excite myself looking at the sexy female pictures in the Playboy magazine. Nothing emotional... Just brief physical satisfaction...

MARY
(suddenly alert, look at him and confront him)
I know, now, why you are testing me... You are
concerned of my health, and you are trying
to justify yourself to get rid of me.

JOSEPH
(bewildered, hold her arm, look at her in the eye)
No... I am not imagining. If I had realized it before your illness, I would have divorced you... I will feel guilty if I divorce you now because of implementing vengeance rather than justice. 'Until Death do us apart' we said. Unfortunately, death is the only peaceful resolution for our departure...
(look at her in the eye)

Were you faithful to me?... Did you
cheat me with other men?...

MARY
(do not answer, turn head away from Joseph,
cover face with hands and begin to cry)

SCENE II
MIDDLE STAGE OF ALZHEIMER'S

Directions
(In the living room, Joseph sits on the chair. He is very depressed. Mary screams from the bedroom)

MARY
No... No... I don't like you... I don't like you... Don't touch me...

Directions
(Bedroom door opens and young companion Judy walks in. She is in her early twenties)

JUDY
Joseph, can you help me. Mary refuses to let me take her clothes off and refuses to take a shower. She is too strong. I can't handle her.

JOSEPH
(quickly get up from chair and rush to the bedroom)
No problem. I will help you.

Directions
(They walk into the bedroom. Mary continues screaming)

MARY
No... I don't like you... I don't want you... Joseph, help me... Joseph, help me...

Directions
(Doorbell rings. Joseph walks out of the bedroom and opens the front door. A man in his late sixties enters. Joseph greets him)

JOSEPH
Hello, Doctor Allen. Good to see you.

Directions
(Doctor Allen ignores Joseph and pushes him aside and quickly walks in. He takes off his coat and hat and gives it to Joseph and walks to the couch and sits. Joseph hangs his coat and sits across from him on the chair)

ALLEN
How are you doing?

JOSEPH
Well, you know how it is… I am exhausted. Now it is the psychological pressure on me… Emotionally, I am falling apart. The caregiver is physically taking care of her.

ALLEN
(look at him with sinister smile)
You know I warned you ten years ago. I told you she has her mother's disease.

JOSEPH
Of course, you know everything!… You are a doctor… Especially, you are an invincible doctor!…

ALLEN
What do you mean?

JOSEPH
Ten years ago, you told me that she had her mother's disease because she was very energetic like her mother. I told you that if lots of energy are the symptom of her illness, then all athletes should have Alzheimer's disease. And then, you diagnosed her disease because her facial skin was much wrinkled. I told you that your diagnosis was very personal because one of our

classmates' facial skin is much wrinkled, and he is an athlete; therefore he should also have Alzheimer's disease. You questioned her social over activity like, stopping people on the street and starting conversation... Your diagnosis was not medical but personal at that time.

ALLEN
I am a doctor, you know!...

JOSEPH
Yes, a typical doctor with 'I know everything' personality. We, the architects, listen to our clients' needs, and then we draw the plans according to their needs. We analyze and evaluate the problems from two point perspective. The doctors and politicians and lawyers and CEO's analyze from one point perspective and evaluate the problem.

ALLEN
Silly, you are like a child...

JOSEPH
I would rather be a child than a self-centered doctor. Your typical doctor's opinion is based on genetics only. You say, 'Your parents had this disease, and you will have the same disease'! Her mother had six siblings, and two of them had Alzheimer's disease and the others did not. Especially, her aunt was as sharp as can be at the age of ninety. It doesn't mean that every child will inherit the same disease of their parents. Why do some children inherit the same genes and some don't?... I don't know the answer... Of course, doctor Allen knows the answer... All I can think of is that nature is not fair... My parents did not have cancer. But my sister and I had cancer.

ALLEN
(uncomfortable, rebut Joseph)
Why do you bother going to doctors if you know better!...

JOSEPH
You are right. I am going to cancel my annual
checkup with my internist doctor.

ALLEN
Which doctors do you see for your medical checkup?

JOSEPH
For my annual medical checkup, I will see President
George W. Bush. At least I can tell him cut the baloney.
We can dispute the presidents, but we can't dispute the
doctors... Because, Doctor Allen knows everything!...

ALLEN
You are childish and cynic!...

JOSEPH
I would rather be childish and cynic
rather than be a hypocrite.

ALLEN
Of course, you didn't do anything about
Mary's medical condition!

JOSEPH
What do you mean 'I didn't do anything'?...
About four years ago, the symptoms of the
early-stage Alzheimer's was apparent.

ALLEN
Did you do anything?...

JOSEPH
Perpetually, I tried to persuade her to see a doctor. She
refused. She was in denial. That is typical symptoms of
Alzheimer's. She would get irritated. I asked you to talk
to her and convince her to see the doctor. You tried once.

She reacted belligerently. You walked out and told me you did't want to get involved. A number of times I asked you to persuade her. I told you that you are a docto and maybe she will listen to you seriously. You did not respond. Her cousin Libby, who is a nurse, was concerned about her. Once in a while she would call and inquire about her health. She was aware of the genetic family condition because Libby's father died of Alzheimer's. Mary was lost and police found her after eight hours wondering in the streets. I called Libby and told her about the deteriorating condition of Mary. Libby told me that she will come to see her, and we can take her to the hospital.

ALLEN
I persuaded Mary to go to the neurologist!

JOSEPH
Yes, in that respect, I give you credit.

ALLEN
I was the one who tricked her to see the neurologist. She had pain in her head. I told her that she may have tumor in her brain and had to see the doctor.

JOSEPH
I know that. She had pain in her neck that escalated towards her head. I believed that the cause of the pain was due to the heavy packages she would carry on her arms when she went shopping for the house... She did everything for the house... Shopping... Cleaning... I must confess, I did nothing...

ALLEN
Of course... You were the "Prince".

JOSEPH
Anyhow... You privately mentioned to the neurologist that Mary has Alzheimer's disease. You told the neurologist

everything about her family's genetic condition. The neurologist examined her and because of her nervous reactions the neurologist thought that she was suffering from Pick's disease and wrote a referral for MRI brain scan. A week later, we went back to the hospital to find out the results of the MRI scan. The neurologist told us the report indicated that Mary did not have any problem. (get up from chair and walk to the bookcase and open the panel and take out medical reports, walk back and sit on the chair and look straight at Allen)
This is the MRI report...
(begin to read)
'Multiplanar and multisequential MRI examination of the orbits, before and after the administration of intravenous gadolinium, was performed. There is no proptosis. The globes are bilaterally unremarkable. The optic nerve sheaths are bilaterally symmetric. The extraocular muscles bilaterally are unremarkable. The retrobulbar fat is unremarkable. There is no intra or extracoronal mass. The paranasal and paracavernous areas are unremarkable. The orbital apices are bilaterally unremarkable. Evaluation of the visualized portions of the brain demonstrates atrophy.
(pause, look at Allen)
Impression number one: Unremarkable MRI examination of the orbits... Number two: Atrophy of the visualized portions of the brain... Number three: Mild atrophy with multiple deep white matter lacunar infarcts... Number four: No mass lesion of the brain is identified.' (glance at Allen)
Of course, you understand the medical terms better than me. Of course, the medical profession prefers to keep their own vocabulary so that patients can't challenge them.

ALLEN
(turn head the other way and ignore Joseph)
You are cynical...

JOSEPH
(take a deep breath, shake head in despair)
The neurologist decided to follow up with the medical examinations and gave a referral for PET scan for Mary. By then, her neck pain discontinued, and she refused to go back for the PET Scan. She was aware of the reason for having the PET Scan done, but she was in denial of her condition. I couldn't convince her. I asked you, again and again, to talk to Mary… Because of her nervous reaction, you refused to get involved.

ALLEN
Doctors can't force the patients.
(tries to exonerate himself)
Do you know about patient's rights?

JOSEPH
Of course, you know everything, doctor Allen, and I know nothing!... Anyhow, there is no way to communicate with you… I was desperate. I said to myself, 'maybe I should call her cousin Libby. Maybe she will help me'. So I called Libby, and she told me to get an appointment for the PET Scan and tell her the date and she will come two days before, and talk to Mary. Libby came and talked to her and tried to convince her. Mary refused.
(sigh)
The appointment was the next day at 2 PM. I called you the night before and asked you to come in and help Libby. You came in the morning and sat down and did not say a word to Mary. Libby was about to give up. I was very frustrated. I realized that I had to convince Mary by challenging her financial security. Believe me, she was always very alert with our finance.

ALLEN
Of course, I know that.

JOSEPH
Of course, you know everything, doctor... Anyhow; I told Mary that she had an appointment in the afternoon with the doctor. If she wouldn't go, in that case, I had to cancel the appointment, and we would lose lots of money. She was surprised and looked at me seriously. 'Why would we lose money?' she asked. I told her that the doctor will charge us the fee because he lost time and money and the insurance company would not reimburse our money. I reiterated that the amount would probably be over a thousand dollars. Mary looked at me seriously. 'I will get ready,' she said and walked into the bedroom... I decided to walk her to the hospital. It was only a twenty minutes' walk, and she would talk to you and her cousin, and that would distract her mind. You walked behind and avoided conversation with her. When she was signed in the admissions office, they told us to wait outside. I told to nurse that my wife is very nervous, and she may get irritated and may walk out. I said it would be better if her cousin, who is a nurse, should stay with her. You and I stayed in the waiting room...

ALLEN
I know that...

JOSEPH
Anyhow... After twenty minutes, Libby came in and sat next to us. She looked depressed. She said, 'Mary almost walked out. I had a very difficult time convincing her to go back to the PET scan'... I am glad that Libby helped me. Otherwise, without her, you and I could do nothing...

ALLEN
You are a cynic... Always negative...

JOSEPH
Anyhow... This is the PET Scan report.
(pick up the report from lap and read)

Examination type: PET BRAIN METABOLIC EVALUATION
Clinical Information: DEMENTIA
Impression: 1. Findings most consistent with Alzheimer's disease.
2. White matter microvascular disease.
Description: CLINICAL INFORMATION: 66-year-old woman with dementia DESCRIPTION: Approximately 40 minutes after the intravenous administration of 11.08 millicuries of Fluorine-18-FDG, a non-contrast CT transmission corrected PET scan of the brain was performed. Serum glucose measured 101 mg/dL before time of injection. No prior study is available for comparison. FINDINGS: There is decrease in glucose metabolism of the parietal lobes bilaterally, right worse than left. To a lesser extent, there is decrease in glucose metabolism in the mesiotemporal lobes bilaterally. Decreased glucose metabolism is also seen in bilateral periventricular matter. The sensorimotor cortices are preserved...
(pause and look at Allen)

ALLEN
Of course... I diagnosed her condition before.

JOSEPH
If you knew it, why did you not tell her and persuade her to see a doctor for an early checkup?!...

MARY
(scream in the bedroom)
I don't like you... I don't want you... Get out... Get out...

ALLEN
(look at Joseph curiously)
What is happening?... What is she doing?...

JOSEPH
Caregiver is giving her a bath. She doesn't want
to be touched by anyone. She has incontinence,
and she has to be washed every day.

ALLEN
How often the caregiver comes?

JOSEPH
She comes eight hours a day, seven days a week.

ALLEN
Of course… You don't want to pay for twenty-four hours
a day… Of course, you don't want to spend your money.
What are you saving your money for? You have no family!…

JOSEPH
Allen… At least listen to my opinion before criticizing me!

ALLEN
What is your opinion?

JOSEPH
She is physically functioning and…

ALLEN
(interrupt)
I want to see her…

JOSEPH
I will bring her.
(quickly get up from the chair and walk into the
bedroom; walk out of the bedroom holding Mary's
hand, direct her to the couch next to Allen)
Mary, your friend came to see you from
Connecticut. Say hello to him.

MARY
(sit down on the couch, look at Allen briefly
and turn to face the opposite way)

ALLEN
How are you doing, Mary?

MARY
(do not respond)

ALLEN
Mary, how is your caregiver? Did she clean you well?

MARY
(look blank at Allen; speech slurred)
Who are you?

JOSEPH
Allen is your friend, remember?... He came all
the way from Connecticut to see you.

ALLEN
How are you feeling? Are you feeling better?...
Are you taking your medication?

MARY
(frustrated)
I am good... I am good

JOSEPH
Allen, don't talk about her illness directly or indirectly.
Sometimes she relates medical questions to her condition.

MARY
(do not respond, look agitated, quickly get up from
the couch and walk towards the bedroom)

JOSEPH
(rush after Mary and grab her arm before
she tries to open the door)
I love you darling.
(lean forward and gently kiss her)
Come back and sit with us. Let us listen to the music.
(hold her hands and guide her to the couch
and gently pull her down to sit)

MARY
(refuse to sit)

JOSEPH
(use short sentences, speak slowly)
Mary darling... Sit down... Make yourself comfortable...
I will turn on the CD... Which is your favorite song?...
Let us listen to Nat King Cole... You need to listen
to soothing songs... (walk to the secretary, put in
a CD in the player and turn it on and a song begins
to play, walk back and sit on the chair next to Allen,
look at Mary and try to start a conversation) Mary
darling, ask Allen about his beloved puppies.

MARY
(mumble)
What puppies?

ALLEN
I know... Mary has aphasia.

JOSEPH
(encourage Mary to concentrate)
Two young boxers are Allen's best friends. Do you
remember Allen cremated the old boxer, and he said
he will bury the ashes with him when he dies?

ALLEN
She is suffering from Agnosia... Joseph, when you looked at her with sadness on your face, she couldn't conceive
(agitated)
Of course, I did save the ashes of my pet... The pet lovers are the only people who love humanity!
(disparaging)
You never had any pets!

JOSEPH
Of course, you are right... Historically speaking, all leaders in the world had pets in their domicile, including in our good old White House... But that did not prevent the first and second World Wars and Vietnam War; and the current and future skirmishes... If you are an animal lover, why do you go to fancy restaurants and eat beef or pork or fish meat? They are animals. Why do you discriminate against then?... Your concept of animal love is same as politicians 'love for freedom and democracy'... You guys are something else!...

ALLEN
You are cynical and stupid...

MARY
(get up from the couch and walk around nervously and murmur incomprehensible words)

JOSEPH
Mary darling, sit down and relax...
(look at Allen and respond to his rebuke)
I admit... I don't deny my lack of abilities. Don't blame me. Blame the nature... I blame my grandfather. He should have married your grandmother so that I would inherit some of your cunning genes.

ALLEN
You are silly and childish

JOSEPH
I know… And I enjoy being childish… Let me tell you the reasons about being a pet lover. Parents love their children. That is human nature. They want to control them and be in charge of their life and direct them to a bright future. Children, most of the time, prefer doing things in their own way. They argue, sometimes disobey, and when they organize their lives, they leave their parents and go away… You and both of your two brothers left your mother. In her old age, she was living by herself until she passed away.

ALLEN
You were not living with your mother when she died!

JOSEPH
I agree… And I regret it… Fortunately, in her case, my sister was taking care of her. As they say, 'sons are sons until they have wives; daughters are daughters until they die'… Anyway, bottom line is that controlling and dominating is a part of human nature. Pets become part of owner's life. Pets never leave their masters until they die…

ALLEN
Dogs are men's best friend…

JOSEPH
Of course, you are right. Dogs are men's best friend as long as you feed them… Men are men's best friends as long as they are fed… If they are not fed, dogs and men bite and kill their masters… In medical school, they did not teach you that humans are a two legged version of our four legged ancestors… Do you remember that your beloved dog Brutus bit you on your neck and the doctor in the hospital told you that if it had bitten you half an inch above, you would be a dead man… Of course, you forgave your pet Brutus and you are going to bury his ashes with you when you die.

ALLEN
You are cynical and stupid...

JOSEPH
I agree... Yet, I would rather be cynical
and stupid than a hypocrite.

MARY
(begin picking up various items in the room and mumble)
This is mine... This mine...
(scream)
This is mine...

JOSEPH
(lean back on the chair; try to divert Allen's attention)
I must admit that I love and respect my ancestors more
than my cousins due to the tragedy of my family.

ALLEN
(alert, wanting to investigate)
Who were your ancestors?

JOSEPH
My ancestors were honest. They always told the
truth. One percent of my cousins are honest and tell
the truth but, unfortunately, they don't survive.

ALLEN
Hello!... I said who are your ancestors?...

JOSEPH
My ancestors kill and steal and when I ask them, 'Why are
you killing and stealing', they tell me the truth and say,
'We are killing and stealing to fill our stomach'... When
I ask my ninety-nine percent of my cousins why are you
killing and stealing, they tell me that they kill and steal
for freedom and democracy; God and country; humanity

and equality... And they give every excuse under the sky... I tell to the ninety-nine percent of my cousins that they are disgusting and despicable sons of bitches and I don't want to see them and don't want to talk to them.

ALLEN
Don't be silly... I asked you, 'Who are
your cousins and ancestors?'...

JOSEPH
(laugh)
OK... I will tell you the truth... Ninety-nine percent of my despicable cousins live in Europe; Asia; Australia; Africa; North and South America; and some of them in the North Arctic region. Unfortunately, one percent of my honest and courageous and outspoken European; Asian; Australian; African; North and South American and the North Arctic cousins don't survive...

ALLEN
Tell me who are your ancestors?

JOSEPH
My beloved and honest ancestors are gorillas and monkeys...

ALLEN
You are crazy...

JOSEPH
I will spend the rest of my life talking to my honest ancestors in the Central Park zoo and Bronx zoo; and in the zoos in London and Paris and Asia, Australia, Africa, North and South America and the North Arctic...

ALLEN
You are silly!

JOSEPH
You are lucky. You did not have the same family problem because your ancestors came from Jupiter, Mars and Venus...

Directions
(door open and companion Judy walk in)

JUDY
(look at Mary)
It is time for lunch.

MARY
(angry, shout)
I don't like you...

JUDY
(walk towards Mary and hold her hand and pull her towards the table and try to sit her on the chair)

MARY
(agitated, scream)
Don't touch me... Don't touch me... I hate you...
(try to release self by pushing companion)

JOSEPH
(get up from the chair and hold Mary's arm)
Darling, you have to have something to eat. Your companion Judy prepared a delicious lunch for you.

Directions
(Joseph pulls the chair and pushes Mary down to sit, then pushes the chair towards the table. Judy opens the door and goes to the kitchen)

ALLEN
How is her appetite?

JOSEPH
She refuses to eat. We have to hand feed her. However, eventually, she finishes her meal. I give her over the counter vitamins... I don't know if the vitamins do any good... Whatever... She has nothing to lose... The medical industry promotes everything. It is a multi-billion dollar industry.

Directions
(Door opens, and the companion walks in with a plate in her hand and sits next to Mary)

JOSEPH
Judy prepared the delicious lunch for you. Thank her...

MARY
(ignore Joseph)

JOSEPH
Take your fork and eat... Pick up the food with the fork...

MARY
(shout)
No... No... I don't want it...

JOSEPH
But darling you have to eat to stay healthy... I will help you...

Directions
(Joseph picks up the food on the plate and brings the fork close to Mary's mouth. Mary refuses to open her mouth. Joseph tries to get her attention)

JOSEPH
OK, I will eat it...
(Joseph brings the fork close to his mouth and pretends to eat)
Wow! So delicious... I love it.

(Joseph brings the fork close to Mary's mouth)
Do you want to eat?...

Directions
(Mary opens her mouth and Joseph puts in the food. Mary begins to chew. Joseph gives the fork to Judy and walks to the chair and sits. Judy waits for Mary to swallow the food, and she picks more food with the fork and puts it in Mary's mouth. Mary begins to chew, and gets up and starts walking around the room)

ALLEN
Does she finish her food?

JOSEPH
Yes, she eventually does. We have to wait until she swallows the food, and wait a while until she takes the next bite.
(watch Mary's movement)
Mary darling, go back to the table and finish your lunch.

JUDY
Mary... Your lunch is ready... Come and eat...

Directions
(Mary walks back to the table. Judy puts food in her mouth. Mary walks away. Judy picks up the plate and follows her around, and when Mary swallows the food, Judy puts more food in Mary's mouth. Mary walks to the table and picks up Allen's handbag. Allen jumps up and grabs his handbag and tries to pull it off her hand. Mary is resistant and angry)

JOSEPH
(try to calm Mary)
Mary... The handbag belongs to Doctor Allen.

MARY
(scream)

No... No... It is mine... It is mine...

JOSEPH
Allen let go your handbag. I will take it.

ALLEN
Are you sure?

JOSEPH
(reach out to the handbag and hold it)
Darling, I will take the bag and I will give it back to you later on... Why you don't go to the bedroom and watch the news...

Directions
(Joseph looks at Judy and makes a facial signal. Judy steps forward and holds Mary with both arms and slowly pulls her away towards the bedroom)

JUDY
(gently)
Mary, I have something for you in the bedroom... Let's go...
(slowly direct Mary into the bedroom)

JOSEPH
(criticize Allen)
You should know that Alzheimer's patients need verbal cues and prompting instead of aggressive attitude towards them. You should use empathy when you communicate with Mary!

ALLEN
Do you think you are a doctor?...

JOSEPH
I attended courses at Alzheimer's Institute for the caregivers.

ALLEN
(agitated, sit down and try to justify self)
You are in denial. Mary needs to be hospitalized.
You can't keep her at home.

JOSEPH
What do you mean by 'hospitalized'?... She had seen
an Alzheimer's specialist. She had medical tests.
Unfortunately, there is no medical solution.

ALLEN
My diagnosis is that she is having psychiatric problem
and my prognosis is that she should go to the
psychiatric hospital for proper medical treatment.

JOSEPH
First of all, she is taking medication to control her
irritability. Irritability is a part of her disease.

ALLEN
There is special ant-psychotic medication
that will stop her agitation.

JOSEPH
(thoughtful, lean back in the chair, hold chin with right hand
and lift face up; lost in thoughts, turn face towards Allen)
Maybe you are right. Maybe I should try the
hospital care... After all, what do I have to lose?
Except, at least five months of my social security
check, which will pay for the hospital fees...

ALLEN
I can write the referral for hospital care.

JOSEPH
Another issue is how I am going to take her to the hospital. She refuses to go to a doctor. I can't reason with her anymore and I can't persuade her.

ALLEN
It is simple. You call 911 and tell them that your wife has a psychiatric problem, and she needs to go to a hospital, and tell them that she is violent, and they should send police officers to control her. Tell them which precinct is in your neighborhood.

JOSEPH
(upset, get up from the chair and slowly walk around in the room, talk to self) Do I have to go through this? Why me?... Why me?...
(slump down on seat)
Doctor Allen, maybe you are right... As they say, 'it is not good to be your own doctor'. Maybe it is right... What a vicious cycle... Experiment and experiment... Medical drug trials are replacing animals with humans... A hopeless journey to the unknown!
(moan)
Oh 'God help me'...

Directions
(stage lights fade)

SCENE III
PLACE THE SAME

Directions
(Joseph is sitting on the chair by the table. He is holding his forehead with his right hand and his arm is resting on the table. He looks desperate, lost in his thoughts. From the bedroom, a mumbling sound is heard. Theoorbell rings, he gets up slowly and walks to the door and opens it. Doctor Allen pushes him aside and walks in. He drops his jacket and his handbag on the couch)

ALLEN
How is Mary?

JOSEPH
(slowly walk back to chair and slouch)
My fears became reality.

ALLEN
Nonsense... You are hallucinating...

JOSEPH
Do you diagnose reality as 'hallucination'?

ALLEN
You are in denial. She is in the third stage of the disease. Deterioration of her physical and cognitive skills are the symptoms of the third stage of Alzheimer's.

JOSEPH
Allen, it is understandable to notice the mental and physical decline in a year. One doesn't need to be a doctor or scientist. Before she checked in to the hospital, she could talk and walk, although her conversation was not normal. After

she was discharged from the hospital, she was physically and mentally debilitated. Now, she can't walk and can't talk.

ALLEN
I have to see her. Where is she?

Directions
(Joseph gets up from the chair and slowly walks into the bedroom. Allen sits down on the couch and curiously looks at the bedroom. Mary enters the living room sitting in a wheelchair. Joseph pushes the wheelchair next to Allen's couch)

ALLEN
(look at Mary curiously)
How are you, Mary?

Directions
(Mary mumbles words; she tries to get up from the chair. Allen tries to help and holds her arm and pulls her up. Joseph reaches out and holds her other arm)

JOSEPH
Allen... She can't walk. We have to keep her in the wheelchair.

ALLEN
I know what I am doing!...

Directions
(Mary takes one step and stumbles. Next step, she loses her balance and collapses. Joseph quickly grabs her by her waist to prevent her hitting the floor)

JOSEPH
(agitated)
I told you doctor, she cannot walk anymore!

Directions
(Joseph and Allen pull her up and put her in the wheelchair. Joseph slumps on the chair. Allen sits on the couch)

JOSEPH
Why the hell did I take her to the psychiatric hospital?!... Why did I comply with the doctor?' prognosis!...

ALLEN
Nonsense!...

JOSEPH
Of course, doctor's sense is the sublime sense... No objections, your honor!... (lean back, exhausted, look at Mary in despair)
Every day, I went to the psychiatric hospital to see her medical condition. I thought I would recognize the progress of her psychological and cognitive skills. The hospital was such a scary place. If the mental patients totally lose their sanity, then the patient wouldn't be aware of the dreadful environment. But the patients like Mary who still had some cognitive skills and could apprehend the horrific environment, for them, living in that condition is worse than living in the prison.

ALLEN
You are always cynical. How can you compare a psychiatric hospital with prison?

JOSEPH
I compare the treatment of the patients... Obviously, patients were insane. They were screaming, running around, harassing each other and provoking the nurses' aides.

ALLEN
What did Mary do?

JOSEPH
Mary was scared. I went to the hospital every day to see her. Each time she saw me she looked at me desperately and said 'Joseph, where are you?' What she really meant was 'Joseph, why did you leave me here?' I would try to calm her down. I would say 'Mary darling you are here temporarily. I will take you back home as soon as the doctor prescribes the right medication for you. Be patient'.
(sigh and close eyes)

ALLEN
Why did you not talk to the doctor?

JOSEPH
Are you kidding me?... Of course, I talked to the doctor. Each time I talked to the doctor, I told him that she was physically and mentally much better before she began taking the medication he prescribed. Also, I told him that the medication he prescribed was banned in England, especially for the patients who are over 62 years old. There were a number of fatalities induced to the Alzheimer's patients who were taking that medication... Of course, our medical industry is untouchable.

ALLEN
What did he say?

JOSEPH
His response was doctors' typical 'I know everything' response. He told me that she is deteriorating due to the advance of her illness.

ALLEN
What did you say?

JOSEPH
I said that anyone can identify the deterioration within a reasonable time period. In her case, in one month, after taking the new prescription in the hospital, she became physically and mentally incapacitated. She couldn't walk and she couldn't talk. It was obvious that these are the side effects of the medication.

ALLEN
Doctor is the specialist, you know!...

JOSEPH
So are the politicians!...

ALLEN
Don't be childish!...

JOSEPH
The bottom line is that he refused to adjust the medication. He told me that I am unrealistic and expecting a miracle.
(take a deep breath and moan)

ALLEN
How long did she stay in the hospital?

JOSEPH
She stayed four weeks.
(look at Allen resentfully)
You came to see her once. You stayed fifteen minutes and walked out. I told you in detail about the side effects of the medication, and you ignored me. You said the same thing!...

ALLEN
What did I say?
Joseph
You said that her deterioration is inevitable; it is not the side effects of the medication. (pause briefly and think)

'Beauty is in the eyes of Doctor Allen'... Actually... The ultimate truth is, 'Beauty is in the eyes of the Almighty Mighty Dollar'... Whatever... No point getting involved with personal opinions. I am telling you what happened.

ALLEN
I am listening...

Joseph
The environment in the psychiatric hospital made her psychological condition worse. She was more agitated and restless. In order to calm her down, they increased the sedatives. When I went to see her, she was in bed, semi-sleeping. In front of her room, two nurses' aides were sitting in the chair to make sure that she wouldn't walk out. She would look at me briefly and say 'Joseph, where are you?', and then, she would look at me desperately. (hold head with both hands and close eyes and moan) Oh, God!... Help me!... What a psychological torture it was!...

ALLEN
How did you resolve the problem?

JOSEPH
There was no resolution. Each time I saw the doctor, I told him to adjust the medication and I told him that I will take her back home. He told me that I can't take her home, and she has to stay another four weeks. I told him that if he does not release Mary, I will talk to my lawyer and proceed with legal action. The doctor thought for a while and said, 'Let me talk to my colleagues', and walked out. I waited in the room for half an hour.

ALLEN
What was the decision?

JOSEPH
The decision was that they could not release her back to home, but they will release her to a nursing home.

ALLEN
What did you do?

JOSEPH
I thought about proceeding with the legal action... I called my lawyer and asked her opinion. She said it would be legally more appropriate to appeal and bring her home from a nursing home rather than the hospital. I thought about the consequences and decided I should bring her home from the nursing home. Otherwise, getting involved with lawyers is as frustrating, like hassling with the doctors or politicians.

ALLEN
(try to divert the criticism of the doctors)
Stop being cynical and stop criticizing the doctors... How did they send Mary to the nursing home?

JOSEPH
(sigh desperately)
Oh, God!... What a day it was!... First, they told me that I don't need to go with her. I told them that she may overreact, and they may have a hard time taking her to the nursing home. They said I can ride with her in the ambulance... Mary was restless and refused to go. I told her that she was being discharged from the hospital, and we were going home. She relaxed. Still, they tied her to the stretcher. I sat next to her in the ambulance and held her hand and repeated that she will eventually be going home. The ambulance traveled along the east river, and I looked out the window and talked to Mary during the infamous journey.

ALLEN
What did you say?... Probably you told her how bad was the service in the hospital and how stupid were the doctors!...

JOSEPH
Whether you like it or not, I tell the truth...
(silent and thoughtful)

ALLEN
(persistent)
What did you talk about with Mary?

JOSEPH
I talked about our memories.
(try to recollect the memories)
I said, 'Do you remember darling, we used to drive down and up the East River to go to midtown or downtown... Do you see that Roosevelt Island and the Randall's Island?... Years ago real estate CEOs were developing the Randall's Island, and they were building condos and coops. I went there hoping I could rent an apartment. I found out that the rent would be twice of my monthly salary'... Those were the days... Days of hopeful expectations...

ALLEN
Don't be cynical... Some smart people achieve their aim and live a good life!

JOSEPH
Of course, you are a doctor and living in a million-dollar mansion in Connecticut... Not to mention that billionaire Mr. Madoff lived in multimillion-dollar mansions... I must admit, it is the survival of the shrewd, not the fittest... Darwin goofed!

ALLEN
Nonsense... Right now, Mr. Madoff is in jail!

JOSEPH
Big deal… The man lived all his life in luxury and plundered money.

ALLEN
Who do you blame?

JOSEPH
Let us analyze in two point perspective like architects.

ALLEN
Stop the 'architect' nonsense. Stop bragging about being an architect…

JOSEPH
Why not? The Supreme Court advocates the federal equal opportunity law… You brag about being a doctor, so I will brag about being an architect…

ALLEN
Who do you blame?

JOSEPH
I blame the human greed… I believe someday doctors will find a cure for Alzheimer's and cancer and other fatal diseases, but they will never find a cure for the destructive greed of humanity. It is an incurable disease… First of all, those who invested in Madoff's Ponzi scheme should have realized that when the economy collapsed and recession began, their investment bonds were still earning high %12 interest. The investors did not question the high-interest rate of the bonds because they were making huge profit… The most important thing is…

ALLEN
What is the most important thing?…

JOSEPH
Did you invest some money in Madoff bonds?

ALLEN
(ignore, turn to face the other way and avoid the question)

JOSEPH
At the beginning of the recession and at the collapse of the stock market, I was worried about you and asked you how you were doing. You said, 'I am doing fine... I am doing fine,' and you accused me of being a cynic. At that time, real estate prices were artificially skyrocketing, and you were satisfied because you had a house worth a million-dollar.

ALLEN
(furious, expression is sullen)
Stop the nonsense

JOSEPH
The most important question is: How the Internal Revenue Service did cope with the Ponzi scheme problem at the beginning?... They check on every citizen's annual income, and tax responsibilities. Every year, I get a letter indicating that I owe fifty or hundred dollars. I checked my annual income and I realized that I made a mistake and sent the IRS the money I owe. Rarely, I do receive a reimbursement check of fifty or one hundred dollars, indicating that I overpaid. I check my records and realize that they were right and I overpaid.

ALLEN
So what?... IRS has the right to check on you!

JOSEPH
I agree. They have to check on every citizen. The point is...
(pause and look at Allen)

During fifty years of Mr. Madoff's Ponzi schemes,
why IRS did not check on his income and taxes
to find about the legality of his business?

ALLEN
Why, you tell me?...

JOSEPH
Let us use our common sense, but not Doctor Allen's sense!

ALLEN
You are childish...

JOSEPH
Probably because Madoff allured billions of dollars of foreign investors and offshore bank investors that contributed to the income of the IRS and Federal Reserve Bank, and they looked the other way... The same thing happened during the great depression...

ALLEN
What happened during the great depression?

JOSEPH
Same thing happened... What they call as 'the roaring twenties' was an artificial stock market growth. The government did not interfere because it brought high hopes to the people and, probably, government also made some profit... The consequence of the irresponsibility of the government and collaboration with the corrupt business caused the great depression and the Second World War. The people paid the high price for their greed and hypocrisy. (look seriously at Allen)
It is the survival of the wicked
(pause, look at Allen, and wait for response)

ALLEN
Cut your bull shit...

JOSEPH
Let us give full credit to the American Institute of Architects and analyze the problems in two point perspective. Let us be realistic... If we elect an architect to be the President of the United States, he can define realistically the cause of the problems by analyzing the issues in two point perspective. Unfortunately, he can't find a solution to the problems because the 'Big Brothers' are in charge of the problems. Politicians analyze the problems in one point perspective to cover up for the 'Big Brothers'. PhD boys and girls in the Ivy League, in Eton College, and in Oxford University teach convoluted 'Official Story' instead of 'Factual History' to the students. The reason why the education system is failing is the deception of the establishment, but not the students' unproductive study!...

ALLEN
(disdainful)
Let me hear your shit!

JOSEPH
Number one
(point one finger at Allen)
Money makes the world go around. The Almighty dollar assassinated the communism; and, former communist countries are going, round and round, around the 'Almighty Mighty Dollar'. Number two:
(point two fingers)
History is based on win or lose conditions. 'Alexander the Conqueror' is recognized as 'Alexander the Great'. If he had lost the war, history would have labeled him as 'Alexander the Barbarian'. We are lucky that our Founding Fathers won the revolution. If they were defeated,

in the present, the British Secret Service and the history books would define them as rebels without a cause and...
(look at Allen with a cunning smile)
Of course, you, as the subject of the
British Empire, would not object...
(start laughing)
Thank heavens, now, we, the citizens, are under the observation of our 'Big Brothers' in Washington, D.C., we can challenge the British.
(serious, briefly pause and think)
If Martin Luther King, Jr., and Malcolm X and other conscientious citizens have lost the civil rights movement, how do you think their cause would be defined?... 'Equal rights movement' or 'Rebellion without a Cause?'

ALLEN
(turn head the other way and ignore)

JOSEPH
(pause and think)
It is a matter of win or lose situation.
(contemptuous)
If you say 'Yes boss, you are right boss', and kiss your bosses' ass, you are 'good'; if you say 'no boss, you are wrong boss' and don't kiss your bosses' ass, you are 'bad'.
(laugh)
Of course, that is why you were always good and successful
(laugh)
You were always delicious 'French fries' because you kissed your bosses ass, and you were never labeled as 'freedom fries'.

ALLEN
(condescend)
Go on with your shit!

JOSEPH
(point three fingers)
Authoritarian regimes are in total control of the society, and officially they do the dirty work if they want to suppress the dissidents. Democratic governments give green light to the organized crime or as they call the 'Mafia', to do the dirty work and eliminate the dissidents. In reality, the organized crime is an unofficial agency of the democratic governments.
(point four fingers)
In reality, NATO is an abbreviation of National Actors Theater Organization. They do wonderful acting, directing and producing political scenarios.

ALLEN
(challenge)
I know why you are always negative... Because you are a communist and atheist!...

JOSEPH
(laugh)
Communism is a dead duck.

ALLEN
(challenge)
Socialists won election in France and Greece!

JOSEPH
(ignore)
Socialists will govern temporarily until the economy improves. Afterward, capitalist will take over. Of course, in medical school, professors don't teach that Socialism is step-sister of capitalism and communism. Socialism is a flip/flop sister. In the medical school they teach that human blood is composed of red blood cells. It is just a theory. The reality is that human blood is composed of green blood cells.

ALLEN
(agitated)
What are you talking about? What do
you mean by 'green blood cells'?

JOSEPH
I will show you the laboratory test results…
(reach out to pants pocket, pull out the pocketbook, take out a dollar bill and begin to wave the dollar)
See!… This is the human blood cell that makes the humanity survive. The people in the former Soviet Union and the communist countries are healthy now, because they transferred 'Almighty green blood cells' to their body from the capitalist blood banks!
(challenge)
The good old United States is the melting pot.
What is the ingredient of the melting pot?
(wave the dollar bill)
The ingredient is the 'Almighty Dollar'. As I told you, not only the immigrants are melted in the pot, but the rest of the world, including the communist countries, are melted. I can see Mr. Gorbachev swimming in the melting pot.

ALLEN
(challenge)
We have ethnics in the United States

JOSEPH
(serious)
Ethnic identity or discrimination in the good old United States is based on the individual bank account and business and political marketing. There are only two ethnic groups in the United States. There are one percent conscientious, honest, courageous and outspoken ethnic Americans and ninety-nine percent Mr. Madoff ethnic Americans… Of course, you belong to the Doctors' ethnic group and live in a million-

dollar mansion. I belong to the ethnic group that depends on the social security retirement pension and struggle to survive... The rest of the world is also same old, same crab... (laugh and continue)
Religions do not change the humanity's quest to kill and steal. Of course, you don't talk about challenging political and social issues because the establishment would kick you out of your million-dollar mansion in Connecticut and you will end up as a homeless man in Washington Heights! Democracy and freedom is a relationship like Caesar and Cleopatra!... And, finally... (look at Allen seriously) Empires rise, and then fall because of corruption. Our American Empire will eventually fall apart, not because of communist and terrorist kiddos, but it will fall apart because of the internal corruption. History repeats itself

ALLEN
(angry)
You are full of bull shit!...

JOSEPH
(laugh)
I prefer to be a bull shit rather than intellectually constipated individual...

ALLEN
(tease and laugh)
Why don't you write a book and be a professor?

JOSEPH
If I write a politically incorrect book, the 'Big Brothers' will make sure that it won't be published and promoted.

ALLEN
(ignore and look the other way, try to divert the issue)
I am not interested in your opinion. I am interested to hear what happened in the nursing home.

JOSEPH
(think for a while)
After traveling north on the East River Drive, we crossed to the Riverdale... It is a nice neighborhood, you know... Next to urban hassle, it is a quiet suburbia... At least it is how it looks like. I am sure there are also some challenges living there. In Manhattan, I walk out of my apartment and walk two blocks to get whatever I need...
(mocking)
How many miles do you have to drive from your million-dollar mansion to a store to get toilet papers?... I mean in case of emergency...

ALLEN
No matter what, I would never live in your Washington Heights... I know... I know... You have the beautiful view of the Hudson River and the beautiful park... Good for you!...

JOSEPH
Wherever we live, let us enjoy the moment... Eventually, we will end up in a nursing home and realize that home is the most important part of our lives... Not the location of our home! (lean back on the chair and sigh)
Anyhow... When the ambulance entered the nursing home, they brought her to the second floor, reserved for the Alzheimer's patients. It was a locked area, so the Alzheimer's patients couldn't walk out of the nursing home. Her room was about eighteen feet by eighteen feet, reserved for two patients. The beds were side by side separated by a curtain. The light was turned off. There was an old woman lying in one bed and constantly mumbling.

ALLEN
How long did you stay with her?

JOSEPH
They told me that they will put her in bed and give her medication and then I can go home.

ALLEN
When did you see her again?

JOSEPH
I went to see her every day.

ALLEN
Nonsense... Why did you have to go and see her every day!... Nursing home takes care of the patients.

JOSEPH
(agitated, mockingly repeat Allen's statement)
'Nursing home takes care of the patients'!... That is doctors' typical prejudice... (look at him angrily) Did you visit her when she was in the nursing home?

ALLEN
(uncomfortable, try to justify self)
When the patients are in a reliable nursing home, there is no need for me to go and interfere with their work. Patients' medical files are sent by the hospitals and the nursing home follows the instructions.

JOSEPH
Exactly... That is the problem... The doctors send their irresponsible prognosis and the nursing home follows the instructions without questioning them...

ALLEN
Joseph, you are stupid!...

JOSEPH
Yes... Yes... I am stupid... I prefer to be
stupid rather than to be a hypocrite...

ALLEN
(ignore him)
I am not interested in your opinion...

JOSEPH
Whatever...
(take a deep breath)
I went to visit her every day to see the progress of her
condition. There was no progress. She was sedated
heavily. They did not want her to walk around and go
to other patient's room. The nursing home personnel
treat the mental patients with frustration... They
kept her sitting in a chair behind a heavy table all day
so that she couldn't get up and wander around. She
would look at me desperately and tell me 'why did you
bring me here, Joseph?... I want to go home!'...
(sorrowful)
After one week, I asked the nurse if they stopped giving
the particular medication prescribed by the doctor in the
hospital. The nurse told me that they cannot make changes
unless the doctor in the nursing home authorizes the change.

ALLEN
What did you do?

JOSEPH
I went home and wrote a letter and explained
the side effects of the prescription and asked the
doctor to stop giving it to marry. Next day I went
to the nursing home and gave the letter to the
nurse and asked him to give it to the doctor.

ALLEN
What did the doctor do?

JOSEPH
I kept on going to the nursing home every day and observed Mary's condition. After two weeks when I realized that there was no improvement, I asked the nurse if they stopped, or at least, adjusted the medication. The nurse said that he gave the letter to the doctor but the doctor did not say anything to him... I was aggravated... I told the nurse that I wanted to see the doctor immediately. The nurse told me that he was in the office reading the files of the patients. I went to his office, introduced myself and wanted to discuss the issue.

ALLEN
What did he say?

JOSEPH
(disgusted)
He claimed that the nurse did not give him my letter and told me that he does not have the time to talk to me. I was very annoyed and told him that if he does not discuss the issue with me now, I will take Mary home immediately.

ALLEN
You couldn't do that!

JOSEPH
When I said 'I was going to take her home', suddenly, the doctor became very uncomfortable.

ALLEN
Why should he be uncomfortable?

JOSEPH
Because, average monthly payment for the nursing homes is seven thousand dollars per month. Losing

a patient would be costly for them. I hope now
you can understand why he was cooperative after
I told him that I will take Mary back home...

> ALLEN
> Did he talk to you?

> JOSEPH
> He told me he will meet me in Mary's room in five minutes.
> I went to her room and waited. He came in and looked
> at Mary and asked the usual questions... 'What day is
> today?'... He pointed at me and said, 'Do you recognize
> this man?'... 'What did you have for breakfast?'...

> ALLEN
> Those are regular questions asked to the Alzheimer's patients
> to probe their mental conditions. What did he tell you?

> JOSEPH
> Nothing! He smiled at me and walked out
> (frustrated, look at Allen furiously)
> He discontinued giving that specific prescription.
> I kept her in the nursing home another week
> and brought her back home yesterday.

> ALLEN
> How did you bring her home?

> JOSEPH
> I went to the nursing home with a taxi and took a caregiver
> with me and brought a wheelchair. The administration
> prepared the release documents and said they will send
> the bill. I had no stamina to discuss with them the amount
> I had to pay out of pocket. I just wanted to take her out
> of the nursing home and bring her back home... Having
> someone breathing at home diminishes my loneliness...
> (thoughtful, look at Allen in dismay)

When I was young, I thought 'drop-dead' was an insult. As I get older, when I realize the nightmare of the old age circumstances, I believe that 'drop-dead' may be a compliment.

ALLEN
(rebuke)
Joseph... Drop dead!...

JOSEPH
Thank you, doctor, for your medical prognosis!...
(look at Allen furiously)
If I remember correctly you removed the feeding tube from Mary's mother to speed the termination of her life. Maybe, Mary agreed with you because she was frustrated and desperate to observe the long-term demise of her mother.

Directions
(Allen and Joseph look at each other with disdain)

ALLEN
Joseph, you are stupid. You should have left Mary in the nursing home permanently. She needs full-time care and you can't do it. Why are you saving your money? You don't have children and Mary's niece, who does not care about her, will inherit the money... Spend your money...

JOSEPH
(resentful)
I may have some money, but do you think I have as much money as Doctor Allen and live in a million-dollar mansion in Connecticut?...

ALLEN
(irritated)
My house does not worth million dollars anymore. Real estate prices plummeted. Democrats are hopeless!...

JOSEPH
Of course, you are a registered Republican!...

ALLEN
(disparage)
You live in a rent controlled apartment
in Washington Heights!...

JOSEPH
Thank goodness... If we didn't have rent control,
then I couldn't even afford to rent your basement...
Unfortunately, the real estate moguls are trying to
abolish the rent control... If that happens, the homeless
shelters will be a thriving Ponzi scheme of the business.

ALLEN
You are always silly and cynical liberal. You guys
are trying to socialize the health care industry!

JOSEPH
How can we dare!... You conservatives control everything.
We thought that a democrat president would reform
the health care system. It turned out that the democrats
were also the concubines of the big business.

ALLEN
What do you mean by concubines? This country
provides equal opportunity to every citizen.

JOSEPH
(resentful)
So they say... Martin Luther King Jr., and Malcolm
X surely got the equal opportunity!!!...

ALLEN
Joseph... I am talking about the health plan!

JOSEPH
That is exactly what I am talking about! They were supposed to improve the Medicare benefits because it does not provide sufficient grant-in-aid for long-term care.

ALLEN
Of course, full financial support by the Medicare will create budget deficit. We can't afford it anymore.

JOSEPH
You are right. The health industry and the doctors will have minimum pay and their standard of living will abate. You will have to leave your million dollar Connecticut mansion and move to the middle-income neighborhood in Washington Heights.

ALLEN
Ridiculous! How would it affect you financially?
Tell me about your financial income,

JOSEPH
First you tell me about your assets and
then I will tell you about mine.
(tease)
Of course, your assets are untouchable. You are a doctor and your high income is due to medical doctors' enormous amount of contribution to health care!...

ALLEN
(ignore Joseph and wait for the information)

JOSEPH
It is very frustrating to prepare for the long-term care for Mary. I checked various sources and discussed it with my lawyer. The middle income is caught in between the rich and the poor. Fortunately, Medicaid is a blessing

for the poor. Rich can handle the financial burden of
the health care. But, guys like me, trying to survive with
social security and have limited assets, are domed.

ALLEN
What do you mean by 'doomed'? Ridiculous statement...

JOSEPH
If I pay Mary's medical and nursing home expenses
out of my pocket, my assets will deplete in four
years. Afterward, she may be eligible for Medicaid,
but I will be eligible for the homeless shelter!

ALLEN
So what do you liberals want to do? Do you want
to make the United States a socialist country?

JOSEPH
Forget about the liberals. Liberals turned out
to be the actors of the 'Big Brothers'.

ALLEN
Childish statement... What do you mean by 'big brothers'?

JOSEPH
I mean... The 'Big Brothers' in the United States
Congress and their superior 'Big Brothers' in the
Stock Exchange, who are the kingmakers.

ALLEN
What are you going to do about it?

JOSEPH
I am a conscientious, honest, courageous and outspoken
citizen. Unfortunately, I can't do anything... I was
hoping that Lady Liberty would do something.
(pause and look at Allen provokingly)

ALLEN
Are you crazy?

JOSEPH
(ignore and annoy him)
I was hoping that my favorite Lady Liberty would swing her torch and smash the heads of the politicians in the United States Congress and in the United Nations. Maybe the politicians would put their act together.

ALLEN
Lady Liberty should smash your head!...

JOSEPH
It is too late. The 'Big Brothers' already smashed my 'politically incorrect' head.

ALLEN
Good for you... What is the market value of your assets?

JOSEPH
The issue is how long can I keep her at home and make her feel secure and comfortable. When is the right time to send her to a nursing home and avoid depleting the financial assets? That is the question!...

ALLEN
You have to send her as soon as possible. She is deteriorating rapidly... Her agitation can be dangerous for you...

JOSEPH
So what!... She can kill me... I don't care... I am tired of living... Life lost its significance...

ALLEN
Listen, Joseph, I am worried and I care about you... You are my childhood friend... Before your mother died, she told me to take care of you. I promised her that I would...

JOSEPH
(subdued, look up, smile sadly, and begin to sing)
Mama, my life is a challenging journey,
The time goes so fast.
Mama, my hopeful dreams were illusion,
Love and peace befit delusion.
Mama I strived for fame and fortune,
I believed in justice and parity,
And fought for freedom and democracy.
Mama nature is not fair,
My health is fading away,
Social justice is rare,
Robber barons are in the limelight,
They are the shining stars.
Mama, I am in the homeless shelter,
Waiting to die,
My soul and body will be forgotten
In the world of the divine.
Mama, please come back from Heaven
Hold your son in your arms
And teach me how to survive
On the life's challenging journey.
Mama, come back to me...

ALLEN
Tell me about your financial situation.

JOSEPH
(wipe tears from face with hand)
I discussed the issue with my lawyer. I told her that in the advanced stage of Alzheimer's, nursing home care will be better for Mary. It may be sooner than I predict. If I do make

personal pay, it will be more than Mary's monthly social security and pension income. So I have to spend our assets. As I told you before, our assets will deplete in four years.

ALLEN
Apply for Medicaid.

JOSEPH
I told you before!... If I apply for Medicaid for Mary, Medicaid will pay for the nursing home; on the other hand, my monthly social security income will make me eligible for the homeless shelter!

ALLEN
(try to be in control, quickly get up from the couch, pick up the coat and walk towards the door) I have to go... Give me a call.
(open the door and walk out)

SCENE IV
PLACE THE SAME

Directions
(Joseph is sitting on the chair next to the table and writing checks for the monthly bills and talking to himself)

JOSEPH
Am I in the golden age or in the golden cage?... Old age is not even a golden cage... It is the burning cage.
(pause and look at the bill)
Another monthly medical and doctors' fees... Shit... When I was young, I used to complain about high taxes... At least I paid the taxes once a year. Now, I am paying the bills every month...

Directions
(Doorbell rings. Joseph gets up, walks to the door and opens. Allen pushes him aside and walks to the couch)

ALLEN
How is Mary?
(take off coat and put it on the couch)

JOSEPH
(close the door and walk back and stand next to Allen, pat him on the shoulder) Good to see you Allen. No matter what, you are an old buddy of mine.

ALLEN
What do you mean by 'no matter what'?

JOSEPH
No matter how much you bug me, still it is good to see you...

ALLEN
Where is Mary?

JOSEPH
Mary is in the bedroom. The caregiver is cleaning her.

Directions
(Mary's angry outcry is heard: 'I don't like you...
I don't want you... No... No... Nooo...)

ALLEN
I want to see Mary.

JOSEPH
(walk to the bedroom and open the door, speak loudly)
Judy... Bring in Mary.
Direction
(Joseph walks back and sits on the chair next to Allen. Allen looks curiously in the bedroom door and waits. The door opens and Mary walks in and Judy follows her. Joseph gets up from the chair and walks to Mary and holds her hand)

JOSEPH
Mary darling, our friend Doctor Allen came to see you. Say 'Hello' to him. It is nice of him to visit and want to see how you are doing.

MARY
(nervous, look furiously)
I am good... I am good...

JOSEPH
Of course, you are good, darling. Have a seat next to Allen.

MARY
(ignore him and begin to walk nervously around the room, begin replacing and picking up small items in the room)

JOSEPH
(look at the caregiver and give instructions)
Judy, bring Mary's meal and put it on the table. Try to persuade her to eat the meal herself. If she resists, then give her meal one spoon at a time and wait until she swallows.

JUDY
(walk inside to the kitchen to bring out Mary's meal)

JOSEPH
(look at Allen)
Physically and mentally, Mary is much better now since she is not taking the medication prescribed in the hospital. Her cognitive skills are better. She is functioning better.

ALLEN
Do you take her out for a walk? Do you use the wheelchair?

JOSEPH
Thank goodness! She is not bedridden anymore. She can walk… Unfortunately, the fact is that she is declining, but not as fast as when she was taking the specific medication which had lethal side effects.

Directions
(Judy walks in and brings food, a glass of water, a fork and knife on a tray and puts the tray on the table)

ALLEN
(question Judy)
How is Mary doing?

JUDY
She is much better since she stopped taking the specific medication.

ALLEN
(uncomfortable, try to impose the judgment of the medical profession)
Doctors always have a valid reason to prescribe the essential medication. It is the physical or DNA condition of the patients that respond positive or negative to the medication. (quickly pick up a coat from the couch and rush to the door to avoid hearing Joseph's opinion. Open the door and walk out without looking back)

JUDY
(walk to the door and close, stop by Joseph and look at him with compassion) Joseph, you are a good man.

Directions
(Joseph looks at Judy affectionately)

JUDY
Joseph, I love you.

Directions
(Judy embraces Joseph and kisses him passionately, and she pulls back; Joseph looks at her intensely, grabs her and kisses her passionately; Mary watches, her face is expressionless; she picks up the fork and knife and stirs the food on the plate. Judy pulls herself away from Joseph and rushes to the bedroom. Joseph is enchanted; slowly he begins walking around the room and talks to himself)

JOSEPH
(loudly)
Oh, God! Is this your blessing or curse?... Am I dreaming... Is this her feminine love or her 'love for daddy'... Why now?... Maybe love and sex is not too late for a man of my age... (pause and think) But she kissed me passionately... Maybe I am not too old for her age... Maybe I still have the

machismo... She will bring a new life to me... This is the beginning of a new life for me. (jubilant) Life goes on... Life is beautiful... Life is beautiful... Thank you, God...

Directions
(Mary continues watching him and nervously stirs the food on the plate with a fork and knife. Her expression is upset. The doorbell rings; Joseph slowly walks to the door and opens; a young man appears)

YOUNG MAN
Is Judy in?

JOSEPH
Excuse me... Who am I talking to?

YOUNG MAN
I am Judy's fiancé. I came to pick her up.

JOSEPH
(perplexed, look back in the bedroom, speak loudly)
Judy... Your boyfriend is here...

JUDY
(heard from the bedroom)
I am coming.

Directions
(Joseph slowly walks to the couch and slumps; bedroom door opens, Judy rushes out towards her fiancé, she kisses him, and they walk out; Joseph gets up from the couch and walks to the door and closes, perplexed and desperate, slowly, Joseph begins wondering around the room and talks to himself)

JOSEPH
Am I dreaming or is this the reality?... What is love?... Is it fiction or is it imagination!! (pause) Doctor Allen was right... I am stupid... I am not a realist... I am a daydreamer!... (pause) Love and hate are relevant to human instincts...
(slowly approach to Mary)

MARY
(look blank at Joseph)

JOSEPH
Mary darling, you know I love you...
(bend over and kiss her)

Directions
(Mary picks up the knife and swings it towards his chest, the knife penetrates into his heart, Joseph moans, looks at Mary, tries to hold on to the table)

JOSEPH
Mary... I am dying... I love you...

Directions
(Joseph loses his balance and falls on the floor and does not move; stage lights dim, Mary slowly gets up from the chair and begins wandering around the room)

MARY
(speak slowly and quietly)
Joseph, where are you?
(pause)
Where are you, Joseph?... I love you... I miss you, Joseph... Don't leave me alone... Joseph, come back to me...
(stage lights dim)

END

www.ingramcontent.com/pod-product-compliance
Lightning Source LLC
LaVergne TN
LVHW041713060526
838201LV00043B/712